Baby Trivia Multiple Choice

See how well you know baby trivia by selecting the correct answers to the following questions. **Scoring:** Each correct answer gets one point. Each incorrect (or skipped) answer loses one point. (Answers on the back cover.)

1. How much did the heaviest surviving baby on record weigh at birth (to the nearest pound)?
a) 18 pounds b) 22 pounds c) 25 pounds d) 29 pounds

2. Who does the voice of the baby in *Look Who's Talking?*
a) Bruce Willis b) Tom Selleck c) Ted Danson d) John Travolta

3. What was the name of the baby who miraculously survived being trapped for several days in a well in 1987?
a) Jeremiah b) Jennifer c) Jason d) Jessica

4. What was the most popular name for American boys in 1900?
a) John b) William c) Michael d) David

5. What was the most popular name for American girls in 1900?
a) Sarah b) Anna c) Emily d) Mary

6. What was the most popular name for American boys in 1998?
a) Matthew b) Brandon c) Nicholas d) Michael

7. What was the most popular name for American girls in 19̄ ̄ ̄
a) Emily b) Sarah c) Ashley d) Brianna

8. How old was the oldest documented mother when she ga
a) 53 b) 63 c) 73 d) 83

9. In what state were the McCaughey septuplets born?
a) Iowa b) Kansas c) Nebraska d) Indiana

10. During which pregnancy trimester does a baby grow the
a) the first b) the second c) the third d) equal for all the

11. For whom is the candy bar Baby Ruth named?
a) Babe Ruth b) President Grover Cleveland's baby dau
c) The daughter of the candy bar's inventor d) nobody

12. Who wrote *The Tales of Peter Rabbit?*
a) Beatrix Potter b) Dr. Seuss c) L.M. Montgomery d) B

Baby Trivia Multiple Choice

See how well you know baby trivia by selecting the correct answers to the following questions. **Scoring:** Each correct answer gets one point. Each incorrect (or skipped) answer loses one point. (Answers on the back cover.)

1. How much did the heaviest surviving baby on record weigh at birth (to the nearest pound)?
a) 18 pounds b) 22 pounds c) 25 pounds d) 29 pounds

2. Who does the voice of the baby in *Look Who's Talking?*
a) Bruce Willis b) Tom Selleck c) Ted Danson d) John Travolta

3. What was the name of the baby who miraculously survived being trapped for several days in a well in 1987?
a) Jeremiah b) Jennifer c) Jason d) Jessica

4. What was the most popular name for American boys in 1900?
a) John b) William c) Michael d) David

5. What was the most popular name for American girls in 1900?
a) Sarah b) Anna c) Emily d) Mary

6. What was the most popular name for American boys in 1998?
a) Matthew b) Brandon c) Nicholas d) Michael

7. What was the most popular name for American girls in 1998?
a) Emily b) Sarah c) Ashley d) Brianna

8. How old was the oldest documented mother when she gave birth?
a) 53 b) 63 c) 73 d) 83

9. In what state were the McCaughey septuplets born?
a) Iowa b) Kansas c) Nebraska d) Indiana

10. During which pregnancy trimester does a baby grow the fastest?
a) the first b) the second c) the third d) equal for all the trimesters

11. For whom is the candy bar Baby Ruth named?
a) Babe Ruth b) President Grover Cleveland's baby daughter
c) The daughter of the candy bar's inventor d) nobody

12. Who wrote *The Tales of Peter Rabbit?*
a) Beatrix Potter b) Dr. Seuss c) L.M. Montgomery d) Buster Brown

Baby Trivia Multiple Choice

See how well you know baby trivia by selecting the correct answers to the following questions. **Scoring:** Each correct answer gets one point. Each incorrect (or skipped) answer loses one point. (Answers on the back cover.)

1. How much did the heaviest surviving baby on record weigh at birth (to the nearest pound)?
a) 18 pounds b) 22 pounds c) 25 pounds d) 29 pounds

2. Who does the voice of the baby in *Look Who's Talking?*
a) Bruce Willis b) Tom Selleck c) Ted Danson d) John Travolta

3. What was the name of the baby who miraculously survived being trapped for several days in a well in 1987?
a) Jeremiah b) Jennifer c) Jason d) Jessica

4. What was the most popular name for American boys in 1900?
a) John b) William c) Michael d) David

5. What was the most popular name for American girls in 1900?
a) Sarah b) Anna c) Emily d) Mary

6. What was the most popular name for American boys in 1998?
a) Matthew b) Brandon c) Nicholas d) Michael

7. What was the most popular name for American girls in 1998?
a) Emily b) Sarah c) Ashley d) Brianna

8. How old was the oldest documented mother when she gave birth?
a) 53 b) 63 c) 73 d) 83

9. In what state were the McCaughey septuplets born?
a) Iowa b) Kansas c) Nebraska d) Indiana

10. During which pregnancy trimester does a baby grow the fastest?
a) the first b) the second c) the third d) equal for all the trimesters

11. For whom is the candy bar Baby Ruth named?
a) Babe Ruth b) President Grover Cleveland's baby daughter
c) The daughter of the candy bar's inventor d) nobody

12. Who wrote *The Tales of Peter Rabbit?*
a) Beatrix Potter b) Dr. Seuss c) L.M. Montgomery d) Buster Brown

Baby Trivia Multiple Choice

See how well you know baby trivia by selecting the correct answers to the following questions. **Scoring:** Each correct answer gets one point. Each incorrect (or skipped) answer loses one point. (Answers on the back cover.)

1. How much did the heaviest surviving baby on record weigh at birth (to the nearest pound)?
a) 18 pounds b) 22 pounds c) 25 pounds d) 29 pounds

2. Who does the voice of the baby in *Look Who's Talking?*
a) Bruce Willis b) Tom Selleck c) Ted Danson d) John Travolta

3. What was the name of the baby who miraculously survived being trapped for several days in a well in 1987?
a) Jeremiah b) Jennifer c) Jason d) Jessica

4. What was the most popular name for American boys in 1900?
a) John b) William c) Michael d) David

5. What was the most popular name for American girls in 1900?
a) Sarah b) Anna c) Emily d) Mary

6. What was the most popular name for American boys in 1998?
a) Matthew b) Brandon c) Nicholas d) Michael

7. What was the most popular name for American girls in 1998?
a) Emily b) Sarah c) Ashley d) Brianna

8. How old was the oldest documented mother when she gave birth?
a) 53 b) 63 c) 73 d) 83

9. In what state were the McCaughey septuplets born?
a) Iowa b) Kansas c) Nebraska d) Indiana

10. During which pregnancy trimester does a baby grow the fastest?
a) the first b) the second c) the third d) equal for all the trimesters

11. For whom is the candy bar Baby Ruth named?
a) Babe Ruth b) President Grover Cleveland's baby daughter
c) The daughter of the candy bar's inventor d) nobody

12. Who wrote *The Tales of Peter Rabbit?*
a) Beatrix Potter b) Dr. Seuss c) L.M. Montgomery d) Buster Brown

Baby Trivia Multiple Choice

See how well you know baby trivia by selecting the correct answers to the following questions. **Scoring:** Each correct answer gets one point. Each incorrect (or skipped) answer loses one point. (Answers on the back cover.)

1. How much did the heaviest surviving baby on record weigh at birth (to the nearest pound)?
a) 18 pounds b) 22 pounds c) 25 pounds d) 29 pounds

2. Who does the voice of the baby in *Look Who's Talking?*
a) Bruce Willis b) Tom Selleck c) Ted Danson d) John Travolta

3. What was the name of the baby who miraculously survived being trapped for several days in a well in 1987?
a) Jeremiah b) Jennifer c) Jason d) Jessica

4. What was the most popular name for American boys in 1900?
a) John b) William c) Michael d) David

5. What was the most popular name for American girls in 1900?
a) Sarah b) Anna c) Emily d) Mary

6. What was the most popular name for American boys in 1998?
a) Matthew b) Brandon c) Nicholas d) Michael

7. What was the most popular name for American girls in 1998?
a) Emily b) Sarah c) Ashley d) Brianna

8. How old was the oldest documented mother when she gave birth?
a) 53 b) 63 c) 73 d) 83

9. In what state were the McCaughey septuplets born?
a) Iowa b) Kansas c) Nebraska d) Indiana

10. During which pregnancy trimester does a baby grow the fastest?
a) the first b) the second c) the third d) equal for all the trimesters

11. For whom is the candy bar Baby Ruth named?
a) Babe Ruth b) President Grover Cleveland's baby daughter
c) The daughter of the candy bar's inventor d) nobody

12. Who wrote *The Tales of Peter Rabbit?*
a) Beatrix Potter b) Dr. Seuss c) L.M. Montgomery d) Buster Brown

Baby Trivia Multiple Choice

See how well you know baby trivia by selecting the correct answers to the following questions. **Scoring:** Each correct answer gets one point. Each incorrect (or skipped) answer loses one point. (Answers on the back cover.)

1. How much did the heaviest surviving baby on record weigh at birth (to the nearest pound)?
a) 18 pounds b) 22 pounds c) 25 pounds d) 29 pounds

2. Who does the voice of the baby in *Look Who's Talking?*
a) Bruce Willis b) Tom Selleck c) Ted Danson d) John Travolta

3. What was the name of the baby who miraculously survived being trapped for several days in a well in 1987?
a) Jeremiah b) Jennifer c) Jason d) Jessica

4. What was the most popular name for American boys in 1900?
a) John b) William c) Michael d) David

5. What was the most popular name for American girls in 1900?
a) Sarah b) Anna c) Emily d) Mary

6. What was the most popular name for American boys in 1998?
a) Matthew b) Brandon c) Nicholas d) Michael

7. What was the most popular name for American girls in 1998?
a) Emily b) Sarah c) Ashley d) Brianna

8. How old was the oldest documented mother when she gave birth?
a) 53 b) 63 c) 73 d) 83

9. In what state were the McCaughey septuplets born?
a) Iowa b) Kansas c) Nebraska d) Indiana

10. During which pregnancy trimester does a baby grow the fastest?
a) the first b) the second c) the third d) equal for all the trimesters

11. For whom is the candy bar Baby Ruth named?
a) Babe Ruth b) President Grover Cleveland's baby daughter
c) The daughter of the candy bar's inventor d) nobody

12. Who wrote *The Tales of Peter Rabbit?*
a) Beatrix Potter b) Dr. Seuss c) L.M. Montgomery d) Buster Brown

Baby Trivia Multiple Choice

See how well you know baby trivia by selecting the correct answers to the following questions. **Scoring:** Each correct answer gets one point. Each incorrect (or skipped) answer loses one point. (Answers on the back cover.)

1. How much did the heaviest surviving baby on record weigh at birth (to the nearest pound)?
a) 18 pounds b) 22 pounds c) 25 pounds d) 29 pounds

2. Who does the voice of the baby in *Look Who's Talking?*
a) Bruce Willis b) Tom Selleck c) Ted Danson d) John Travolta

3. What was the name of the baby who miraculously survived being trapped for several days in a well in 1987?
a) Jeremiah b) Jennifer c) Jason d) Jessica

4. What was the most popular name for American boys in 1900?
a) John b) William c) Michael d) David

5. What was the most popular name for American girls in 1900?
a) Sarah b) Anna c) Emily d) Mary

6. What was the most popular name for American boys in 1998?
a) Matthew b) Brandon c) Nicholas d) Michael

7. What was the most popular name for American girls in 1998?
a) Emily b) Sarah c) Ashley d) Brianna

8. How old was the oldest documented mother when she gave birth?
a) 53 b) 63 c) 73 d) 83

9. In what state were the McCaughey septuplets born?
a) Iowa b) Kansas c) Nebraska d) Indiana

10. During which pregnancy trimester does a baby grow the fastest?
a) the first b) the second c) the third d) equal for all the trimesters

11. For whom is the candy bar Baby Ruth named?
a) Babe Ruth b) President Grover Cleveland's baby daughter
c) The daughter of the candy bar's inventor d) nobody

12. Who wrote *The Tales of Peter Rabbit?*
a) Beatrix Potter b) Dr. Seuss c) L.M. Montgomery d) Buster Brown

Baby Trivia Multiple Choice

See how well you know baby trivia by selecting the correct answers to the following questions. **Scoring:** Each correct answer gets one point. Each incorrect (or skipped) answer loses one point. (Answers on the back cover.)

1. How much did the heaviest surviving baby on record weigh at birth (to the nearest pound)?
a) 18 pounds b) 22 pounds c) 25 pounds d) 29 pounds

2. Who does the voice of the baby in *Look Who's Talking?*
a) Bruce Willis b) Tom Selleck c) Ted Danson d) John Travolta

3. What was the name of the baby who miraculously survived being trapped for several days in a well in 1987?
a) Jeremiah b) Jennifer c) Jason d) Jessica

4. What was the most popular name for American boys in 1900?
a) John b) William c) Michael d) David

5. What was the most popular name for American girls in 1900?
a) Sarah b) Anna c) Emily d) Mary

6. What was the most popular name for American boys in 1998?
a) Matthew b) Brandon c) Nicholas d) Michael

7. What was the most popular name for American girls in 1998?
a) Emily b) Sarah c) Ashley d) Brianna

8. How old was the oldest documented mother when she gave birth?
a) 53 b) 63 c) 73 d) 83

9. In what state were the McCaughey septuplets born?
a) Iowa b) Kansas c) Nebraska d) Indiana

10. During which pregnancy trimester does a baby grow the fastest?
a) the first b) the second c) the third d) equal for all the trimesters

11. For whom is the candy bar Baby Ruth named?
a) Babe Ruth b) President Grover Cleveland's baby daughter
c) The daughter of the candy bar's inventor d) nobody

12. Who wrote *The Tales of Peter Rabbit?*
a) Beatrix Potter b) Dr. Seuss c) L.M. Montgomery d) Buster Brown

What's the Next Line?

Below are excerpts from popular songs that include the word "baby."
See if you can remember the next line to each song. **Scoring:** One point
for each correct answer plus two points if you know the tune well enough
to sing the song. (Answers on back cover.)

1. "Baby face, . . ."

_____

2. "Yes, sir, that's my baby,"

_____

3. "Maybe, baby, you'll be true."

_____

4. "So keep on rock'n me, baby,"

_____

5. "Love shack, baby! Love shack, . . ."

_____

6. "Come on, baby, and rescue me."

_____

7. "Ooh, baby love, my baby love,"

_____

8. "You must have been a beautiful baby,"

_____

9. "Baby, baby, I'm taken with the notion,"

_____

10. "Ain't got nothin' but love, babe,"

_____

11. "Baby's good to me, you know, she's happy as can be, . . ."

_____

12. "Babe,"

_____

What's the Next Line?

Below are excerpts from popular songs that include the word "baby."
See if you can remember the next line to each song. **Scoring:** One point
for each correct answer plus two points if you know the tune well enough
to sing the song. (Answers on back cover.)

1. "Baby face, . . ."

_____

2. "Yes, sir, that's my baby,"

_____

3. "Maybe, baby, you'll be true."

_____

4. "So keep on rock'n me, baby,"

_____

5. "Love shack, baby! Love shack, . . ."

_____

6. "Come on, baby, and rescue me."

_____

7. "Ooh, baby love, my baby love,"

_____

8. "You must have been a beautiful baby,"

_____

9. "Baby, baby, I'm taken with the notion,"

_____

10. "Ain't got nothin' but love, babe,"

_____

11. "Baby's good to me, you know, she's happy as can be, . . ."

_____

12. "Babe,"

_____

What's the Next Line?

Below are excerpts from popular songs that include the word "baby."
See if you can remember the next line to each song. **Scoring:** One point
for each correct answer plus two points if you know the tune well enough
to sing the song. (Answers on back cover.)

1. "Baby face, . . ."

_____

2. "Yes, sir, that's my baby,"

_____

3. "Maybe, baby, you'll be true."

_____

4. "So keep on rock'n me, baby,"

_____

5. "Love shack, baby! Love shack, . . ."

_____

6. "Come on, baby, and rescue me."

_____

7. "Ooh, baby love, my baby love,"

_____

8. "You must have been a beautiful baby,"

_____

9. "Baby, baby, I'm taken with the notion,"

_____

10. "Ain't got nothin' but love, babe,"

_____

11. "Baby's good to me, you know, she's happy as can be, . . ."

_____

12. "Babe,"

_____

What's the Next Line?

Below are excerpts from popular songs that include the word "baby."
See if you can remember the next line to each song. **Scoring:** One point
for each correct answer plus two points if you know the tune well enough
to sing the song. (Answers on back cover.)

1. "Baby face, . . ."

_____

2. "Yes, sir, that's my baby,"

_____

3. "Maybe, baby, you'll be true."

_____

4. "So keep on rock'n me, baby,"

_____

5. "Love shack, baby! Love shack, . . ."

_____

6. "Come on, baby, and rescue me."

_____

7. "Ooh, baby love, my baby love,"

_____

8. "You must have been a beautiful baby,"

_____

9. "Baby, baby, I'm taken with the notion,"

_____

10. "Ain't got nothin' but love, babe,"

_____

11. "Baby's good to me, you know, she's happy as can be, . . ."

_____

12. "Babe,"

_____

What's the Next Line?

Below are excerpts from popular songs that include the word "baby."
See if you can remember the next line to each song. **Scoring:** One point
for each correct answer plus two points if you know the tune well enough
to sing the song. (Answers on back cover.)

1. "Baby face, . . ."

_____

2. "Yes, sir, that's my baby,"

_____

3. "Maybe, baby, you'll be true."

_____

4. "So keep on rock'n me, baby,"

_____

5. "Love shack, baby! Love shack, . . ."

_____

6. "Come on, baby, and rescue me."

_____

7. "Ooh, baby love, my baby love,"

_____

8. "You must have been a beautiful baby,"

_____

9. "Baby, baby, I'm taken with the notion,"

_____

10. "Ain't got nothin' but love, babe,"

_____

11. "Baby's good to me, you know, she's happy as can be, . . ."

_____

12. "Babe,"

_____

What's the Next Line?

Below are excerpts from popular songs that include the word "baby."
See if you can remember the next line to each song. **Scoring:** One point
for each correct answer plus two points if you know the tune well enough
to sing the song. (Answers on back cover.)

1. "Baby face, . . ."

_____

2. "Yes, sir, that's my baby,"

_____

3. "Maybe, baby, you'll be true."

_____

4. "So keep on rock'n me, baby,"

_____

5. "Love shack, baby! Love shack, . . ."

_____

6. "Come on, baby, and rescue me."

_____

7. "Ooh, baby love, my baby love,"

_____

8. "You must have been a beautiful baby,"

_____

9. "Baby, baby, I'm taken with the notion,"

_____

10. "Ain't got nothin' but love, babe,"

_____

11. "Baby's good to me, you know, she's happy as can be, . . ."

_____

12. "Babe,"

_____

What's the Next Line?

Below are excerpts from popular songs that include the word "baby."
See if you can remember the next line to each song. **Scoring:** One point
for each correct answer plus two points if you know the tune well enough
to sing the song. (Answers on back cover.)

1. "Baby face, . . ."

_____

2. "Yes, sir, that's my baby,"

_____

3. "Maybe, baby, you'll be true."

_____

4. "So keep on rock'n me, baby,"

_____

5. "Love shack, baby! Love shack, . . ."

_____

6. "Come on, baby, and rescue me."

_____

7. "Ooh, baby love, my baby love,"

_____

8. "You must have been a beautiful baby,"

_____

9. "Baby, baby, I'm taken with the notion,"

_____

10. "Ain't got nothin' but love, babe,"

_____

11. "Baby's good to me, you know, she's happy as can be, . . ."

_____

12. "Babe,"

_____

What's the Next Line?

Below are excerpts from popular songs that include the word "baby."
See if you can remember the next line to each song. **Scoring:** One point
for each correct answer plus two points if you know the tune well enough
to sing the song. (Answers on back cover.)

1. "Baby face, . . ."

_____

2. "Yes, sir, that's my baby,"

_____

3. "Maybe, baby, you'll be true."

_____

4. "So keep on rock'n me, baby,"

_____

5. "Love shack, baby! Love shack, . . ."

_____

6. "Come on, baby, and rescue me."

_____

7. "Ooh, baby love, my baby love,"

_____

8. "You must have been a beautiful baby,"

_____

9. "Baby, baby, I'm taken with the notion,"

_____

10. "Ain't got nothin' but love, babe,"

_____

11. "Baby's good to me, you know, she's happy as can be, . . ."

_____

12. "Babe,"

_____

Famous Parent/Child Pairs

For this game, you need to figure out the famous parent/child pair for each description. **Scoring:** For each correct answer, you get one point. For each wrong or skipped question, you lose one point. (Answers on the back cover.)

1. The mother starred in *The Wizard of Oz* while her daughter starred in the Broadway show *Cabaret.*

———————————————
———————————————

2. The father starred in *Apocalypse Now.* His sons are also actors, one of whom starred in *Platoon* while the other starred in *The Breakfast Club.* Name all three of them.

———————————————
———————————————
———————————————
———————————————

3. This father and son are two of the most successful reggae singers ever.

———————————————
———————————————

4. The father was a successful folk rock singer in the sixties; his son now leads his own rock band.

———————————————
———————————————

5. Name the only father and son to both serve as president of the United States.

———————————————
———————————————

6. What mother and daughter became famous as a country music duo?

———————————————
———————————————

7. The father's signature song was "Imagine," while his son scored with "Too Late for Goodbyes."

———————————————
———————————————

8. The father played George Castanza's father on *Seinfeld,* while his son starred in *There's Something about Mary.*

———————————————
———————————————

9. When this father-son pair played for the Seattle Mariners, they made history as the only father and son to both play in the major leagues at the same time. In addition, the son has won four consecutive Gold Glove awards.

———————————————
———————————————

10. The father is a former president of the United States, while his sons are governors of Florida and Texas. Name all three of them.

———————————————
———————————————
———————————————

Famous Parent/Child Pairs

For this game, you need to figure out the famous parent/child pair for each description. **Scoring:** For each correct answer, you get one point. For each wrong or skipped question, you lose one point. (Answers on the back cover.)

1. The mother starred in *The Wizard of Oz* while her daughter starred in the Broadway show *Cabaret*.

_____

_____

2. The father starred in *Apocalypse Now*. His sons are also actors, one of whom starred in *Platoon* while the other starred in *The Breakfast Club*. Name all three of them.

_____

_____

_____

3. This father and son are two of the most successful reggae singers ever.

_____

_____

4. The father was a successful folk rock singer in the sixties; his son now leads his own rock band.

_____

_____

5. Name the only father and son to both serve as president of the United States.

_____

_____

6. What mother and daughter became famous as a country music duo?

_____

_____

7. The father's signature song was "Imagine," while his son scored with "Too Late for Goodbyes."

_____

_____

8. The father played George Castanza's father on *Seinfeld*, while his son starred in *There's Something about Mary*.

_____

_____

9. When this father-son pair played for the Seattle Mariners, they made history as the only father and son to both play in the major leagues at the same time. In addition, the son has won four consecutive Gold Glove awards.

_____

_____

10. The father is a former president of the United States, while his sons are governors of Florida and Texas. Name all three of them.

_____

_____

_____

Famous Parent/Child Pairs

For this game, you need to figure out the famous parent/child pair for each description. **Scoring:** For each correct answer, you get one point. For each wrong or skipped question, you lose one point. (Answers on the back cover.)

1. The mother starred in *The Wizard of Oz* while her daughter starred in the Broadway show *Cabaret*.

_____

_____

2. The father starred in *Apocalypse Now*. His sons are also actors, one of whom starred in *Platoon* while the other starred in *The Breakfast Club*. Name all three of them.

_____

_____

_____

_____

3. This father and son are two of the most successful reggae singers ever.

_____

_____

4. The father was a successful folk rock singer in the sixties; his son now leads his own rock band.

_____

_____

5. Name the only father and son to both serve as president of the United States.

_____

_____

6. What mother and daughter became famous as a country music duo?

_____

_____

7. The father's signature song was "Imagine," while his son scored with "Too Late for Goodbyes."

_____

_____

8. The father played George Castanza's father on *Seinfeld,* while his son starred in *There's Something about Mary.*

_____

_____

9. When this father-son pair played for the Seattle Mariners, they made history as the only father and son to both play in the major leagues at the same time. In addition, the son has won four consecutive Gold Glove awards.

_____

_____

10. The father is a former president of the United States, while his sons are governors of Florida and Texas. Name all three of them.

_____

_____

_____

_____

Famous Parent/Child Pairs

For this game, you need to figure out the famous parent/child pair for each description. **Scoring:** For each correct answer, you get one point. For each wrong or skipped question, you lose one point. (Answers on the back cover.)

1. The mother starred in *The Wizard of Oz* while her daughter starred in the Broadway show *Cabaret*.

_____

_____

2. The father starred in *Apocalypse Now*. His sons are also actors, one of whom starred in *Platoon* while the other starred in *The Breakfast Club*. Name all three of them.

_____

_____

_____

_____

3. This father and son are two of the most successful reggae singers ever.

_____

_____

4. The father was a successful folk rock singer in the sixties; his son now leads his own rock band.

_____

_____

5. Name the only father and son to both serve as president of the United States.

_____

_____

6. What mother and daughter became famous as a country music duo?

_____

_____

7. The father's signature song was "Imagine," while his son scored with "Too Late for Goodbyes."

_____

_____

8. The father played George Castanza's father on *Seinfeld,* while his son starred in *There's Something about Mary.*

_____

_____

9. When this father-son pair played for the Seattle Mariners, they made history as the only father and son to both play in the major leagues at the same time. In addition, the son has won four consecutive Gold Glove awards.

_____

_____

10. The father is a former president of the United States, while his sons are governors of Florida and Texas. Name all three of them.

_____

_____

_____

Famous Parent/Child Pairs

For this game, you need to figure out the famous parent/child pair for each description. **Scoring:** For each correct answer, you get one point. For each wrong or skipped question, you lose one point. (Answers on the back cover.)

1. The mother starred in *The Wizard of Oz* while her daughter starred in the Broadway show *Cabaret.*

_____

_____

2. The father starred in *Apocalypse Now.* His sons are also actors, one of whom starred in *Platoon* while the other starred in *The Breakfast Club.* Name all three of them.

_____

_____

_____

3. This father and son are two of the most successful reggae singers ever.

_____

_____

4. The father was a successful folk rock singer in the sixties; his son now leads his own rock band.

_____

_____

5. Name the only father and son to both serve as president of the United States.

_____

_____

6. What mother and daughter became famous as a country music duo?

_____

_____

7. The father's signature song was "Imagine," while his son scored with "Too Late for Goodbyes."

_____

_____

8. The father played George Castanza's father on *Seinfeld,* while his son starred in *There's Something about Mary.*

_____

_____

9. When this father-son pair played for the Seattle Mariners, they made history as the only father and son to both play in the major leagues at the same time. In addition, the son has won four consecutive Gold Glove awards.

_____

_____

10. The father is a former president of the United States, while his sons are governors of Florida and Texas. Name all three of them.

_____

_____

_____

Famous Parent/Child Pairs

For this game, you need to figure out the famous parent/child pair for each description. **Scoring:** For each correct answer, you get one point. For each wrong or skipped question, you lose one point. (Answers on the back cover.)

1. The mother starred in *The Wizard of Oz* while her daughter starred in the Broadway show *Cabaret*.

_____

_____

2. The father starred in *Apocalypse Now*. His sons are also actors, one of whom starred in *Platoon* while the other starred in *The Breakfast Club*. Name all three of them.

_____

_____

_____

3. This father and son are two of the most successful reggae singers ever.

_____

_____

4. The father was a successful folk rock singer in the sixties; his son now leads his own rock band.

_____

_____

5. Name the only father and son to both serve as president of the United States.

_____

_____

6. What mother and daughter became famous as a country music duo?

_____

_____

7. The father's signature song was "Imagine," while his son scored with "Too Late for Goodbyes."

_____

_____

8. The father played George Castanza's father on *Seinfeld,* while his son starred in *There's Something about Mary.*

_____

_____

9. When this father-son pair played for the Seattle Mariners, they made history as the only father and son to both play in the major leagues at the same time. In addition, the son has won four consecutive Gold Glove awards.

_____

_____

10. The father is a former president of the United States, while his sons are governors of Florida and Texas. Name all three of them.

_____

_____

_____

Famous Parent/Child Pairs

For this game, you need to figure out the famous parent/child pair for each description. **Scoring:** For each correct answer, you get one point. For each wrong or skipped question, you lose one point. (Answers on the back cover.)

1. The mother starred in *The Wizard of Oz* while her daughter starred in the Broadway show *Cabaret.* _____

_____

2. The father starred in *Apocalypse Now.* His sons are also actors, one of whom starred in *Platoon* while the other starred in *The Breakfast Club.* Name all three of them. _____

_____

_____

3. This father and son are two of the most successful reggae singers ever. _____

_____

4. The father was a successful folk rock singer in the sixties; his son now leads his own rock band. _____

_____

5. Name the only father and son to both serve as president of the United States. _____

_____

6. What mother and daughter became famous as a country music duo? _____

_____

7. The father's signature song was "Imagine," while his son scored with "Too Late for Goodbyes." _____

_____

8. The father played George Castanza's father on *Seinfeld,* while his son starred in *There's Something about Mary.* _____

_____

9. When this father-son pair played for the Seattle Mariners, they made history as the only father and son to both play in the major leagues at the same time. In addition, the son has won four consecutive Gold Glove awards. _____

_____

10. The father is a former president of the United States, while his sons are governors of Florida and Texas. Name all three of them. _____

_____

_____

Famous Parent/Child Pairs

For this game, you need to figure out the famous parent/child pair for each description. **Scoring:** For each correct answer, you get one point. For each wrong or skipped question, you lose one point. (Answers on the back cover.)

1. The mother starred in *The Wizard of Oz* while her daughter starred in the Broadway show *Cabaret*.

_____

_____

2. The father starred in *Apocalypse Now*. His sons are also actors, one of whom starred in *Platoon* while the other starred in *The Breakfast Club*. Name all three of them.

_____

_____

_____

3. This father and son are two of the most successful reggae singers ever.

_____

_____

4. The father was a successful folk rock singer in the sixties; his son now leads his own rock band.

_____

_____

5. Name the only father and son to both serve as president of the United States.

_____

_____

6. What mother and daughter became famous as a country music duo?

_____

_____

7. The father's signature song was "Imagine," while his son scored with "Too Late for Goodbyes."

_____

_____

8. The father played George Castanza's father on *Seinfeld,* while his son starred in *There's Something about Mary.*

_____

_____

9. When this father-son pair played for the Seattle Mariners, they made history as the only father and son to both play in the major leagues at the same time. In addition, the son has won four consecutive Gold Glove awards.

_____

_____

10. The father is a former president of the United States, while his sons are governors of Florida and Texas. Name all three of them.

_____

_____

_____

Baby Name Scramble

For this game, unscramble the following list of baby names. Whoever gets the most names correct in three minutes wins. Just so you know, all of these names are in the top twenty-five names for boys and girls. (Answers on the back cover.)

LEMICHA   _____

LYTAIKN   _____

DOIMASN   _____

PHOTERCISRH   _____

NABRINA   _____

VIDAD   _____

TANOJHAN   _____

BANYTRIT   _____

SIXELA   _____

STINUJ   _____

HAZYACR   _____

JASESIC   _____

COLASIHN   _____

NAGEM   _____

NRISTIACH   _____

KAITENHER   _____

RAHSA   _____

THEWAMT   _____

JOBCA   _____

HANNAH   _____

Baby Name Scramble

For this game, unscramble the following list of baby names. Whoever gets the most names correct in three minutes wins. Just so you know, all of these names are in the top twenty-five names for boys and girls. (Answers on the back cover.)

LEMICHA   _____

LYTAIKN   _____

DOIMASN   _____

PHOTERCISRH   _____

NABRINA   _____

VIDAD   _____

TANOJHAN   _____

BANYTRIT   _____

SIXELA   _____

STINUJ   _____

HAZYACR   _____

JASESIC   _____

COLASIHN   _____

NAGEM   _____

NRISTIACH   _____

KAITENHER   _____

RAHSA   _____

THEWAMT   _____

JOBCA   _____

HANNAH   _____

Baby Name Scramble

For this game, unscramble the following list of baby names. Whoever gets the most names correct in three minutes wins. Just so you know, all of these names are in the top twenty-five names for boys and girls. (Answers on the back cover.)

LEMICHA   _____

LYTAIKN   _____

DOIMASN   _____

PHOTERCISRH   _____

NABRINA   _____

VIDAD   _____

TANOJHAN   _____

BANYTRIT   _____

SIXELA   _____

STINUJ   _____

HAZYACR   _____

JASESIC   _____

COLASIHN   _____

NAGEM   _____

NRISTIACH   _____

KAITENHER   _____

RAHSA   _____

THEWAMT   _____

JOBCA   _____

HANNAH   _____

Baby Name Scramble

For this game, unscramble the following list of baby names. Whoever gets the most names correct in three minutes wins. Just so you know, all of these names are in the top twenty-five names for boys and girls. (Answers on the back cover.)

LEMICHA   _____

LYTAIKN   _____

DOIMASN   _____

PHOTERCISRH   _____

NABRINA   _____

VIDAD   _____

TANOJHAN   _____

BANYTRIT   _____

SIXELA   _____

STINUJ   _____

HAZYACR   _____

JASESIC   _____

COLASIHN   _____

NAGEM   _____

NRISTIACH   _____

KAITENHER   _____

RAHSA   _____

THEWAMT   _____

JOBCA   _____

HANNAH   _____

Baby Name Scramble

For this game, unscramble the following list of baby names. Whoever gets the most names correct in three minutes wins. Just so you know, all of these names are in the top twenty-five names for boys and girls. (Answers on the back cover.)

LEMICHA   _____

LYTAIKN   _____

DOIMASN   _____

PHOTERCISRH   _____

NABRINA   _____

VIDAD   _____

TANOJHAN   _____

BANYTRIT   _____

SIXELA   _____

STINUJ   _____

HAZYACR   _____

JASESIC   _____

COLASIHN   _____

NAGEM   _____

NRISTIACH   _____

KAITENHER   _____

RAHSA   _____

THEWAMT   _____

JOBCA   _____

HANNAH   _____

Baby Name Scramble

For this game, unscramble the following list of baby names. Whoever gets the most names correct in three minutes wins. Just so you know, all of these names are in the top twenty-five names for boys and girls. (Answers on the back cover.)

LEMICHA   _____

LYTAIKN   _____

DOIMASN   _____

PHOTERCISRH   _____

NABRINA   _____

VIDAD   _____

TANOJHAN   _____

BANYTRIT   _____

SIXELA   _____

STINUJ   _____

HAZYACR   _____

JASESIC   _____

COLASIHN   _____

NAGEM   _____

NRISTIACH   _____

KAITENHER   _____

RAHSA   _____

THEWAMT   _____

JOBCA   _____

HANNAH   _____

Baby Name Scramble

For this game, unscramble the following list of baby names. Whoever gets the most names correct in three minutes wins. Just so you know, all of these names are in the top twenty-five names for boys and girls. (Answers on the back cover.)

LEMICHA   _____

LYTAIKN   _____

DOIMASN   _____

PHOTERCISRH   _____

NABRINA   _____

VIDAD   _____

TANOJHAN   _____

BANYTRIT   _____

SIXELA   _____

STINUJ   _____

HAZYACR   _____

JASESIC   _____

COLASIHN   _____

NAGEM   _____

NRISTIACH   _____

KAITENHER   _____

RAHSA   _____

THEWAMT   _____

JOBCA   _____

HANNAH   _____

Baby Name Scramble

For this game, unscramble the following list of baby names. Whoever gets the most names correct in three minutes wins. Just so you know, all of these names are in the top twenty-five names for boys and girls. (Answers on the back cover.)

LEMICHA   _____

LYTAIKN   _____

DOIMASN   _____

PHOTERCISRH   _____

NABRINA   _____

VIDAD   _____

TANOJHAN   _____

BANYTRIT   _____

SIXELA   _____

STINUJ   _____

HAZYACR   _____

JASESIC   _____

COLASIHN   _____

NAGEM   _____

NRISTIACH   _____

KAITENHER   _____

RAHSA   _____

THEWAMT   _____

JOBCA   _____

HANNAH   _____